Ketogenic Diet For Beginners

The Complete Ketogenic Diet Guide to Lose
Weight Without Giving Up your Favorite Meals

Amelia Green

Table of Content

Introduction

Thank you for purchasing **Ketogenic Diet For Beginners: The Complete Ketogenic Diet Guide to Lose Weight Without Giving Up your Favorite Meals**

The ketogenic diet began as a low-carbohydrate dietary plan aimed at reducing seizures in patients who did not respond to medication, especially in children. Very low carbohydrate diets have been used since the 1920s for this very purpose.

Since the sixties, these diets have been widely used for the treatment of obesity, but also in the presence of other pathological conditions such as diabetes, polycystic ovary syndrome, acne: it was in fact observed that, in addition to acting on convulsions, they produced positive effects on body fat, blood sugar, cholesterol and hunger levels.

The ketogenic diet has, therefore, increasingly established itself as a diet to lose weight, which exploits the consequences for the body of the reduction of carbohydrates and the increased consumption of fats, not for therapeutic purposes, but to stimulate weight loss.

BREAKFAST

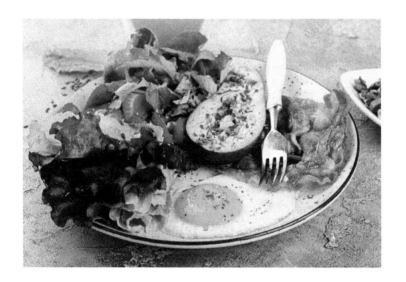

Baked Omelet with Bacon

Preparation Time: 5 minutes

Cooking Time: 30 minutes

Servings: 1

Ingredients:

- 4 eggs

- 140 g diced bacon

- 85 g butter

- 60 g fresh spinach

- 1 tbsp. l finely chopped fresh onions (to taste)

- salt and pepper

Directions:

1. Preheat the oven to 400 ° F. Oil one small baking dish (per serving).

2. Fry the bacon and spinach in the remaining oil.

3. In another bowl, whisk the eggs until it's foamy. Mix the bacon and spinach, gradually adding the fat remaining after frying the products.

4. Then add finely chopped onions. Flavor the dish with salt and pepper.

5. Put the mixture into a baking sheet then bake for at least 20 minutes or until golden brown.

6. Recover the dish and let it cool for a few minutes. After that, you can serve.

Nutrition: Carbohydrates: 12 g Fats: 72 g Proteins: 21 g Calories: 737

Sandwiches With Salad

Preparation Time: 5 minutes

Cooking Time: 0 minutes

Servings: 1

Ingredients:

- 50 g Roman salad

- 15 g Butter

- 30 g Cheese of Eden cheese or other cheese (to your taste)

- 0.5 pcs Avocado

- 1 pc cherry tomato

Directions:

1. Rinse the lettuce leaves thoroughly and use them as a base for the filling.

2. Oil the leaves, chop the cheese, avocado, and tomato and place on the leaves.

Nutrition: Fats: 34 g Proteins: 10 g Carbohydrates: 3 g Calories: 374

Keto Omelet with Mushrooms

Preparation Time: 5 minutes

Cooking Time: 10 minutes

Servings: 1

Ingredients:

- 3 eggs

- 30 g butter for frying

- 30 g (60 ml) grated cheese

- 1/5 onion

- 3 pcs. mushrooms

- salt and pepper

Directions:

1. Break the eggs then put the contents into a small bowl.

2. Add salt and pepper to taste.

3. Beat the eggs with a fork until a uniform foam is formed.

4. In a pan, heat a piece of butter, and as soon as the butter has melted, pour the egg mixture into the pan.

5.   When the mixture begins to harden and fry, and the eggs on top will still be liquid, sprinkle them with cheese, mushrooms, and onions (to taste).

6.   Take a spatula and gently pry the edges of the omelet on one side, and then fold the omelet in half. As soon as the dish begins to take a golden brownish tint, remove the pan from the stove then place the omelet on a plate.

Nutrition: Carbohydrates: 5 g Fats: 44 g Proteins: 26 g Kcal: 649

KETO BREAD

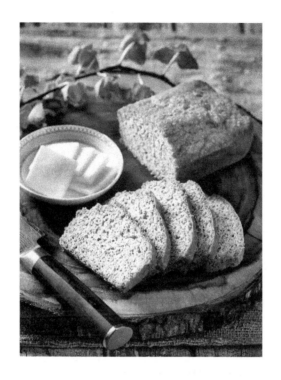

Lemon & Rosemary Low Carb Shortbread

Preparation Time: 5 minutes

Cooking Time: 20 min

Serving: 6

Ingredients:

- 6 tablespoons margarine

- 2 cups almond flour

- 1/3 cup granulated Splenda (or other granulated sugar)

- 1 tablespoon naturally ground lemon get-up-and-go

- 4 teaspoons crisp pressed lemon juice

- 1 teaspoon vanilla concentrate

- 2 teaspoons rosemary*

- 1/2 teaspoon preparing pop

- 1/2 teaspoon preparing powder

Directions:

1. In a huge blending bowl, measure out 2 cups of almond flour, 1/2 tsp. heating powder and 1/2 tsp. preparing pop. Include 1/3 cup Splenda, or other granulated sugar to the blend. Put in a safe spot.

2.   Zest your lemon with a Microplane until you have 1 Tbsp. lemon get-up-and-go. Squeeze a large portion of the lemon to get 4tsp lemon juice.

3.   In the microwave, liquefy 6 Tbsp. of margarine and afterward include 1 tsp. vanilla concentrate.

4.   Transfer your almond flour and sugar to a little blending bowl. Put your spread, lemon get-up-and-go, lemon squeeze, and slashed rosemary into the now vacant huge blending bowl. Include your almond flour once more into the wet blend gradually, mixing as you go. Continue blending until all the almond flour is included back.

5.   Wrap the mixture firmly in cling wrap.

6.   Place the enveloped batter by the cooler for 30 minutes, or until hard.

7.   Preheat your stove to 350F, evacuate your batter, and unwrap it.

8.   Cut your batter in ~1/2" increases with a sharp blade. In the event that this blade isn't sharp, it will cause the batter to disintegrate. On the off chance that the mixture is as yet

disintegrating, that implies it needs additional time in the cooler.

9.   Grease a treat sheet with SALTED margarine and spot your treats onto it.

Nutrition: Cal: 100, Carbs: 2g Fiber: 4.5 g, Fat: 10 g, Protein: 2g, Sugars: 4 g.

Iranian Flat Bread (Sangak)

Preparation Time: 3 hours

Cooking Time: 15 minutes

Servings: 6

Ingredients:

- 4 cups almond flour

- 2 1/2 cups warm water

- 1 Tbsp. instant yeast

- 12 tsp. sesame seeds

- Salt to taste

Directions:

1. Add 1 tbsp. yeast to 1/2 cup warm water using a bowl and allow to stand for 5 minutes.

2. Add salt add 1 cup of water. Let stand for 10 minutes longer.

3. Put one cup of flour at a time, and then add the remaining water.

4. Knead the dough and then shape into a ball and let stand for 3 hours covered.

5. Preheat the oven to 480F.

6. By means of a rolling pin, roll out the dough, and divide into 6 balls.

7. Roll each ball into 1/2 inch thick rounds.

8. Place a parchment paper on the baking sheet and place the rolled rounds on it.

9. With a finger, make a small hole in the middle and add 2 tsp sesame seeds in each hole.

10. Bake for 3 to 4 minutes, then flip over and bake for 2 minutes more.

11. Serve.

High-Fiber Bran Bread:

Preparation time: 1 hour

Cooking time: 2 hours

Servings: 8

Ingredients:

- 355 ml warm water

- 2 tablespoons (16 g) nonfat dry milk

- 2 tablespoons (28 ml) vegetable oil, for example, canola

- 2 tablespoons (40 g) molasses

- 2 tablespoons (40 g) nectar

- 9 g salt

- 281.3 g Stone Ground Whole Grain Whole Wheat

Graham Flour

- 156.3 g Bread Flour

- 1 cup (125 g) Wheat Bran, Unprocessed

- 8 g Fast-Rise Yeast

Directions:

1. Spot ingredients in bread dish as per producer's

bearings. Select entire wheat and begin the machine.

2. Yield: 682.5-g loaf

3.   Set machine on the mixture cycle. When the cycle is processed, structure batter into a loaf and spot in lubed 22.5 cm x 12.5 cm x 7.5-cm container.

4.   Enable the second ascent to top of container and heat in 350F stove for about 35 - 40 minutes or until moment read thermometer embedded in focus enrolls at any rate 190.

Nutrition: Cal: 321, Carbs: 4 g Fiber: 9 g, Fat: 12 g, Protein: 28 g, Sugars: 3 g.

German Dark Rye Bread:

Preparation time: 1 hour

Cooking time: 3 hours

Servings: 8

Ingredients:

- 263 ml warm water

- 1/4 cup (80 g) nectar

- 2 tablespoons (28 g) margarine, diminished,

- 3.1 g caraway seeds (discretionary)

- 6 g salt

- 2 cups (250 g) All-Purpose, Unbleached Naturally White Flour

- 15.6 g unsweetened cocoa powder

- 125 g Stone Ground Whole Grain Rye Flour

- 14 g Vital Wheat Gluten

- 5 g Fast-Rise Yeast

Directions:

1.   Spot ingredients in bread skillet as per producer's headings. Select the entire wheat cycle and begin the machine.

2.   Yield: 682.5-g loaf

3. For a significantly simpler approach to make Dark Rye, utilize (16 ounces Caraway Rye Bread Mix.

4. For 682.5-g loaf, pour 1 cup (240 ml) water in your bread machine, alongside 2 tablespoons (28 g) spread/margarine or (28 ml) vegetable oil, 3 tablespoons (60 g) molasses, and 3 tablespoons (24 g) unsweetened cocoa powder. Include the bread blend and yeast parcel. Utilize the entire wheat bread setting.

Nutrition: Cal: 213, Carbs: 2 g Fiber: 11 g, Fat: 13 g, Protein: 27 g, Sugars: 1 g.

Low Carb Flax Bread

Preparation Time: 10 minutes

Cooking Time: 24 min

Serving: 8

Ingredients:

- 200 g ground flax seeds

- 1/2 cup psyllium husk powder

- 1 tablespoon heating powder

- 1 1/2 cups soy protein separate

- 1/4 cup granulated Stevia

- 2 teaspoons salt

- 7 enormous egg whites

- 1 enormous entire egg

- 3 tablespoons margarine

- 3/4 cup water

Directions:

1. Preheat broiler to 350 degrees F.

2. Mix phylum husk, heating powder, protein disengage, sugar, and salt together in a bowl.

3.	In a different bowl, blend egg, egg whites, margarine, and water together.

4.	Slowly add wet fixings to dry fixings and consolidate.

5.	Grease your bread dish with spread or splash.

6.	Add blend to bread dish

7.	Bake 15-20 minutes until set.

Nutrition: Cal: 20, Carbs: 3.5 g, Fiber: 8.5 g, Fat: 13 g, Protein: 10g, Sugars: 5 g.

Gluten-Free Potato Soy Bread:

Preparation Time: 10 minutes

Cooking Time: 45 minutes

Servings: 5

Ingredients:

- Three huge eggs or proportional egg substitute

- 5 ml juice vinegar

- 45 ml of olive oil

- 112.5 g pureed potatoes

- 315 ml warm water

- 125 g Whole Grain Multi-Purpose Baking Mix

- 125 g Stone Ground Whole Grain Brown Rice Flour

- 130 g custard flour or potato starch

- 62.5 g Soy Flour

- 28 g thickener

- 45 g stuffed light or dim dark colored sugar

- 3 g salt

- 10 g Fast-Rise Yeast

Directions:

1.   Whisk eggs, vinegar, and olive oil together in a huge bowl. Rush in pureed potatoes and water and fill the bread dish. Begin machine on batter cycle. Include preparing the blend, rice flour, potato starch, soy flour, thickener, darker sugar, and salt. Include yeast.

2.   When the cycle is finished, stop the machine. At that point, go to prepare the process. Or on the other hand, cautiously spoon mixture into lubed 22.5 cm x12.5 cm x 7.5-cm loaf skillet and smooth top with a spatula. Enable the second ascent to the top of the dish and heat in 350F broiler for about 45 to 50 minutes or until moment read thermometer embedded in focus enrolls at any rate 190F. Turn out onto wire rack to cool.

3.   Yield: a 455-g loaf.

Nutrition: Cal: 230, Carbs: 4g Fiber: 9.5 g, Fat: 10 g, Protein: 5g, Sugars: 3 g.

Honey Mustard Bread:

Preparation time: 1 hour

Cooking time: 2 hours

Servings: 5

Ingredients:

- 120 ml warm water

- 187.5 g Bread Flour

- 62.5 g Stone Ground Whole Grain Whole Wheat Graham Flour

- 3.2 g nonfat dry milk

- 50 g nectar

- 3 g salt

- 60 ml chicken juices

- 26.3 g Dijon mustard

- 1 g clipped chives

- 4 g Fast-Rise Yeast

Directions:

1. For the two plans: Place all ingredients in bread skillet as indicated by producer's bearings. Select the entire wheat cycle and begin the machine.

2.   Yield: 455-g standard or 682.5-g huge loaf

3.   Set machine on the mixture cycle. When the cycle is processed, structure batter into a loaf and spot in lubed 22.5 cm x 12.5 cm x 7.5-cm container.

4.   Enable the second ascent to top of container and heat in 350F stove for about 35 - 40 minutes or until moment read thermometer embedded in focus enrolls at any rate 190.

Nutrition: Cal: 289, Carbs: 3 g Fiber: 9 g, Fat: 12 g, Protein: 28 g, Sugars: 3 g.

Potato Wheat Soy Bread:

Preparation time: 4 hours

Cooking time: 4 hours

Servings: 8

Ingredients:

- 6 g salt

- 15 g pressed light or dim dark colored sugar

- 10 g Fast-Rise Yeast

- 165 ml soy or 2 percent milk

- 125 g Stone Ground Whole Grain Whole Wheat Graham Flour

- 93.8 g Bread Flour

- 31.3 g Soy Flour

- 56.3 g pureed potatoes

Directions:

1. Spot ingredients in the bread dish as indicated by the maker's headings. Select the entire cycle or entire wheat cycle and light outside layer setting. At that point, begin the machine.

2. Yield: a 455-g loaf

3.   Set machine on batter cycle. When a process is finished, structure mixture into a loaf and spot in lubed 22.5 cm x 12.5 cm x 7.5 cm dish.

4.   Enable the second ascent to the top of the skillet and prepare in 350F stove for about 35 to 40 minutes or until moment read thermometer embedded in focus enrolls at any rate 190F.

5.   Turn out to wire rack to cool.

Nutrition: Cal: 218, Carbs: 2 g Fiber: 9 g, Fat: 10 g, Protein: 8 g, Sugars: 2 g.

Pumpernickel Bread:

Preparation time: 2 hours

Cooking time: 2 hours

Servings: 6

Ingredients:

- 175 ml warm water

- 125 g Bread Flour

- 41.7 g Stone Ground Whole Grain Whole Wheat Graham Flour

- 83.3 g Stone Ground Whole Grain Rye Flour

- 8 g nonfat dry milk

- 24.5 g sugar

- 6 g salt

- 24.5 g margarine, diminished

- 18 g Whole Grain Yellow Corn Meal Mix, Self-Rising

- 13 g unsweetened cocoa powder

- 30 g molasses

- 0.6 g moment espresso powder

- 2.1 g caraway seeds

- 6 g Fast-Rise Yeast

Directions:

1. Place ingredients in bread skillet as indicated by the producer's guidelines. Select the entire wheat cycle and begin the machine.

2. Yield: 455-g standard or 682.5-g huge loaf

3. When manipulating some portion of the process is finished, stop the engine. Reset to batter cycle to consider the second work and then allow the mixture to rise.

4. When the second cycle is finished, isolate the combination into four or two segments. Put aside to ascend until mixture is inside 1 inch (2.5 cm) of top of jars or shape, around 30 minutes.

5. Heat in 375F broiler for about 30 to 35 minutes or until moment read thermometer embedded in focus enlists in any event 190F. Turn out to wire rack to cool. Cut into rounds to serve.

Nutrition: Cal: 216, Carbs: 1 g Fiber: 3 g, Fat: 10 g, Protein: 13 g, Sugars: 1 g.

Garlic and Sun-Dried Tomato Bread:

Preparation time: 2 hours

Cooking time: 3 hours

Servings: 8

Ingredients:

- 12 sun-dried tomatoes

- 175 ml bubbling water

- 60 ml warm water

- 4.5 g salt

- 7.5 ml vegetable oil, for example, canola

- 62.5 g Stone Ground Whole Grain Whole Wheat

Graham Flour

- 312.5 g Bread Flour

- 8 g sugar

- 1 g dried rosemary,

- 3 g garlic powder

- 8 g Fast-Rise Yeast

Directions:

1. Fill a medium bowl with 3/4 cup (175 ml) bubbling

water, at that point splash 8 sun-dried tomatoes in water for

10 minutes or until plumped. Put aside 4 remaining sun-dried tomatoes for the last advance.

2.   Cut tomatoes into little pieces. Include the 1;4 cups (60 ml) warm water to depleted tomato water to make 1 cup (235 ml) fluid.

3.   Spot plumped tomatoes, 1 cup (235 ml) tomato/water fluid, salt, oil, flours, sugar, rosemary, garlic powder, and yeast in the bread machine. Spot remaining sun-dried tomatoes over dry ingredients. Select the fundamental cycle, utilizing light outside layer alternative, and begin the machine.

4.   Yield: One I-pound (455-g) loaf

Nutrition: Cal: 321, Carbs: 1 g Fiber: 12 g, Fat: 10 g, Protein: 21 g, Sugars: 1 g.

Saucy Apple Bread

Preparation time: 2 hours

Cooking time: 2 hours

Servings: 6

Ingredients:

- 120 ml apple juice

- 167 g Bread Flour

- 109 g Stone Ground Whole Grain Whole Wheat

Graham Flour

- 6 g salt

- 22 g yogurt (plain)

- 22 g nectar

- 1.2 ml vanillas concentrate

- 30 g pecans, slashed

- One egg, beaten

- 81.6 g unsweetened applesauce

- 50 g Granny Smith apple, unpeeled and diced

- 3 g Fast-Rise Yeast

Directions:

1.   Place ingredients in bread dish as indicated by maker's headings. Select the essential cycle and begin the machine.

2.   Yield: 455-g ordinary or 682.5-g enormous loaf

3.   Set machine on batter cycle. When a process is finished, structure mixture into a loaf and spot in lubed 22.5 cm x 12.5 cm x 7.5 cm container.

4.   Enable the second ascent to the top of the skillet and prepare in 350F broiler for about 35 to 40 minutes or until moment read thermometer embedded in focus enrolls at any rate 190F.

5.   Turn out to wire rack to cool.

Nutrition: Cal: 312, Carbs: 2.9 g Fiber: 5 g, Fat: 12 g, Protein: 58 g, Sugars: 1 g.

Low Carb Focaccia Bread

Preparation Time: 10 minutes

Cooking Time: 25 min

Serving: 12

Ingredients:

- 1 cup almond flour

- 1 cup flaxseed feast

- 7 enormous eggs

- 1/4 cup olive oil

- 1 1/2 tablespoons heating powder

- 2 teaspoons minced garlic

- 1 teaspoon salt

- 1 teaspoon rosemary

- 1 teaspoon red bean stew chips

Directions:

1. Preheat your broiler to 350F.

2. In a blending bowl, join all your dry fixings and blend well.

3.   Start including your garlic and 2 eggs one after another, blending in with a hand blender to get a mixture sort of consistency.

4.   Add your olive oil last, blending it well until everything is joined. The more aerated the hitter turns into, the more "cushy" your bread will turn into.

5.   Put every one of your fixings into a lubed 9x9 heating dish, smooth out with a spatula.

6.   Bake for 25 minutes.

7.   Let cool for 10 minutes and expel from the lubed heating dish.

8.   Cut into squares and cut the squares down the middle. Add whatever you'd prefer to the center!

Nutrition: Cal: 50, Carbs: 2.5 g, Fiber: 4.5 g, Fat: 8 g, Protein: 8g, Sugars: 3 g.

KETO PASTA

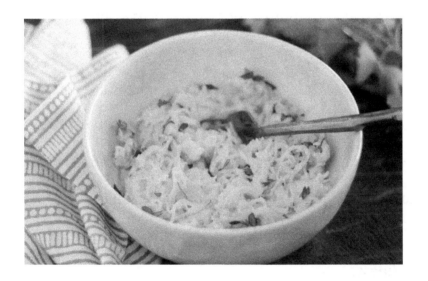

Egg Pasta

Preparation time: 40 minutes

Cooking time: 25 minutes

Servings: 1

Ingredients

- One large egg yolk

- A cup of low moisture Mozzarella cheese (shredded)

Directions

1. Put the mozzarella into a point and microwave for 1-2 minutes

2. Take the cheese out and stir until fully melted. If cheese appears to have lumps, microwave for 1 more minute.

3. Let cool for 1-3 minutes before adding the egg (to avoid scrambling it).

4. Stir the yolk and cheese mixture until you have a smooth yellow dough.

5. Line a flat surface with a piece of parchment paper and place your dough on it.

6.	Cover the dough with another parchment and use a rolling pin to flatten and thin out. Continue thinning it out until your dough is less than a quarter inch thick.

7.	Remove the top parchment and cut your dough into long, thin strips.

8.	When you are done,place your strips of dough (with bottom piece of parchment paper) on a flat tray or plate and put into the refrigerator to dry out.

9.	Put in the pasta and let cook for 1 minute. You have to be careful not to overcook if or the pasta will begin to break and melt.

10.	Once the pasta is ready, sieve and run under cold water to cool.

11.	Use your hands to gently peel apart any strands that might be glued together.

Nutrition: Calories: 358 Total Fat: 22g Carbs: 3g Protein: 33g

Paleo Cabbage Slaw

Preparation time: 10 minutes

Cooking time: 15 minutes

Serves: 6

Ingredients:

- 1 cup Paleo Mayo (here)

- 2 to 3 tablespoons agave

- 2 tablespoons apple cider vinegar

- 2 teaspoons celery seed

- Salt

- Freshly ground black pepper

- 1 small to medium cabbage, spiralized

Directions:

1. In a small bowl, combine the mayonnaise, agave, apple cider vinegar, and celery seed. Stir well and season with salt and pepper.

2. In a large bowl, spoon the dressing over the cabbage noodles and toss to combine.

3. Refrigerate for at least 15 to 20 minutes before serving.

Nutrition: Calories 194 Fat 13g, Protein 11g, Carbs 2g, Fiber 21g

Palmini Low-Carb Pasta

Preparation time: 5 minutes

Cooking time: 2 minutes

Servings: 1

Ingredients:

- A tablespoon of butter

- Two (2) tablespoons of parmesan cheese (shredded)

- Four (4) fresh basil leaves

- A quarter teaspoon of black pepper.

- A can of palmini linguine (drained and rinsed)

- A quarter teaspoon of salt

Directions:

1. Boil the drained and rinsed palmini in a pot of water for five minutes on medium heat.

2. Drain the palmini.

3. Put the cheese and butter in a bowl and microwave for 1 minute or until fully melted.

4. Sprinkle some salt on the parmini and pour it into the melted cheese, add pepper and serve with a few leaves of fresh basil.

Nutrition: Calories: 201 Total Fat: 14g Carbs: 12g Protein: 9g

Salmon and Avocado Pesto Zucchini Noodles

Preparation time: 10 minutes

Cooking time: 7 minutes

Servings: 4

Ingredients

- Skinless wild salmon (4-ounce)

- Black pepper and salt

- Pesto (1 tablespoon)

- Large zucchini (1)

- Avocado (.25 of 1)

- Cherry tomatoes (3)

Directions:

1.   Warm the oven in advance to 425 Fahrenheit.

2.   Prepare a baking tray with a layer of parchment baking paper.

3.   Trim the noodles in a processor using the D blade. Slice the avocado and slice the tomatoes into halves.

4. Place the salmon on the paper and sprinkle using the pepper and salt.

5. Bake until the salmon flakes and are opaque (8-10 min.).

6. In the meantime, toss the pesto with the zucchini noodles until they're covered.

7. Arrange the noodles in a pasta dish and garnish using avocados, tomatoes, and salmon before serving.

Nutrition: Calories: 165 Fat: 28 g Carb: 2 g Protein: 13 g

Mushroom Pasta with Shirataki Noodles

Preparation time: 10 minutes

Cooking time: 20 minutes

Servings: 2

Ingredients

- Shirataki noodles (2 packages)

- Butter (2 tablespoons)

- Garlic (2 cloves)

- Assorted mushrooms (3 cups)

- Almond flour (1 teaspoon)

- Dried parsley (1 pinch)

- Thick cream (.75 of 1 tub)

- Salt (.25 teaspoon)

- Pepper (.25 teaspoon)

- Olive oil

- For the Garnish: Freshly chopped parsley

Directions:

1. Toss the shirataki noodles into a dry frying pan using the medium heat temperature setting. Continue to cook until

you hear a whistling sound, indicating the excess moisture leaving the noodles. Transfer to the countertop to cool.

2.   Toss the butter into the skillet with the garlic, and sauté for approximately 1 minute or until fragrant.

3.   Pour in the oil and add the mushrooms. Sauté for another five minutes, occasionally stirring until the mushrooms are golden in color. Transfer the mushrooms from the pan, leaving the oil behind.

4.   Add the almond flour, salt, pepper, dried parsley, and cream. Stir and simmer to combine.

5.   Lastly, toss the mushrooms and shirataki noodles into the skillet and combine. Serve right away.

Nutrition: Calories: 432 Fat: 22 g Carb: 2 g Protein: 21 g

Sausage Alfredo with Zucchini Noodles

Preparation time: 10 minutes

Cooking time: 7 minutes

Servings: 4

Ingredients

- Bulk hot Italian sausage (12 ounces)

- Butter (2 tablespoons)

- Cloves of garlic (3 minced)

- Heavy whipping cream (1 cup)

- Salt and pepper (as desired)

- Medium zucchini (2)

- Freshly grated parmesan (.5 cup)

Directions:

1.   In a large frying pan using the medium temperature heat setting, brown the sausage 5 to 8 minutes. Transfer to a bowl, leaving a portion of grease in the skillet.

2.   Toss the butter into the pan to melt and add the garlic. Sauté for about 1 minute.

3.   Pour in the cream. Once boiling, reduce the heat setting to low until thickened (5 to 8 min.). Whisk frequently.

4. Whisk in the parmesan, pepper, and salt. Mix the sausage back in and whisk to combine.

5. Spiralize the zucchini noodles into a microwave-safe bowl and cook using the high setting for 2 minutes or until just tender.

6. Divide into four plates and top with the sausage alfredo. Serve immediately for the best results.

Nutrition: Calories: 432 Fat: 26 g Carb: 2 g Protein: 13 g

Keto Carbonara Pasta

Preparation time: 10 minutes

Cooking time: 15 minutes

Servings: 1

Ingredients:

- 150 grams of bacon

- One large egg yolk

- A packet of miracle noodles

- A cup of heavy whipping cream

- Two (2) tablespoons of parmesan cheese

- 60 grams of chicken breast

Directions:

1.   Dice the chicken and Chicken in separate plates.

2.   Set both to cook separately in a frying pan for 5 minutes.

3.   Note: Do not let the bacon become crispy.

4.   Put parmesan cheese and egg yolk in a small bowl and mix until it forms a paste.

5.   Pour the cheese mixture into a frying pan and put on medium heat.

6. Add half the amount of cream and mix until a smooth creamy paste is formed.

7. Add the other half of the cream,bacon and chicken. Stir until fully coated.

8. Dry fry miracle noodles in another pan for 10 minutes, stirring continuously so it doesn't stick or burn.

9. Mix the noodles with sauce and serve.

Nutrition: Calories: 580 Total Fat: 50g Carbs: 5g Protein: 27g

Pesto Shirataki Noodles–Vegan

Preparation time: 10 minutes

Cooking time: 7 minutes

Servings: 4

Ingredients

- Shirataki noodles (2–8-ounce packages)

- Fresh basil (2 cups packed)

- Minced garlic (1 clove)

- Pine nuts (.25 cup)

- Nutritional yeast (.25 cup)

- Salt (1 pinch)

- Olive or pistachio oil (.25 cup)

Directions:

1. Drain and rinse the shirataki noodles thoroughly. Boil for two to three minutes or microwave for one minute.

2. Combine the remainder of the fixings in a food processor, drizzling in olive oil while the motor is running.

3. Mix the pesto with the prepared noodles and serve.

Nutrition: Calories: 432 Fat: 22 g Carb: 2 g Protein: 21 g

Creamy Zoodles

Preparation time: 2 minutes

Cooking time: 3 minutes

Servings: 1

Ingredients:

- Three (3) cloves of minced garlic

- Two (2) tablespoons of butter

- Two (2) medium zucchini

- A quarter teaspoon salt to taste

- A quarter teaspoon pepper

- A quarter cup of parmesan cheese

Directions:

1.   Wash your zucchini then cut it to strands using a spiralizer or vegetable peeler then set aside. If done right, your zucchini should come out like spaghetti strands. I mean, that's the point right?

2.   Put a large pan on medium heat. Put the butter in to melt and then add minced garlic. Stir fry the garlic until it starts to appear translucent. If you know you have an affinity

for burning things, please be attentive so the garlic doesn't get burnt.

3.   Add your zucchini strands and stir fry for three minutes. Make sure to taste your noodle strands to check how tender they are as zucchini cooks really fast. Try not to "taste" till it finishes.

4.   Bring down the pan, add salt, pepper and parmesan cheese, stir until well combined and serve..

Nutrition: Calories: 100 Total Fat: 4g Carbs: 4g Protein: 4g

Salmon Pasta

Preparation time: 10 minutes

Cooking time: 7 minutes

Servings: 4

Ingredients

- Coconut oil (2 tablespoons)

- Smoked salmon (8 ounces)

- Zucchini (2)

- Keto-friendly mayo (.25 cup)

Directions:

1. Melt the oil in a skillet using the med-high temperature setting.

2. Add the salmon and sauté for 2-3 minutes or until lightly browned.

3. Prepare the zucchini using a peeler or spiralizer to make the noodle-like strands. Toss into the skillet and sauté for 1-2 minutes.

4. Mix in the mayo before serving.

Nutrition: Calories: 327 Fat: 21 g Carb: 3 g Protein: 21 g

KETO CHAFFLE

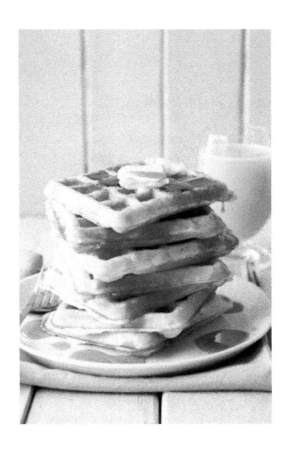

Duckfila Chaffles

Preparation Time: 5 minutes

Cooking Time: 20 minutes

Servings: 2

Ingredients:

- Seared duck breast pieces – 1

- Pickle juice – 4 tablespoons

- Parmigiano cheese – 4 tablespoons

- Pork rinds – 2 tablespoons

- Butter – 1 teaspoon

- Flaxseed (ground) – 1 teaspoon

- Salt (as desired)

- Black pepper powder – 1/4 teaspoon

- For bun

- Shredded mozzarella – 1 cup

- Egg – 1

- Butter extract – 1/4 teaspoon

- Stevia glycerite – 4 drops

Directions:

1. Cut half- inch duck pieces and soak in pickle juice for one hour minimum

2. Pre-heat air fryer

3. Mix all other duck ingredients in one bowl

4. Drain pickle juice and add duck into bowl

5. Let duck cook for 6 min on each side at 400°

6. Mix all bun ingredients together in one bowl

7. Place in waffle maker to cook for about 4 min

8. Sandwich the cooked duck between the buns

Nutrition: Calories 139 Total Fat 4.6 g Total Carbs 2.5 g Sugar 6.3 g Fiber 0.6 g Protein 3.8 g

Smoked ham Cheese Chaffles

Preparation Time: 5 minutes

Cooking Time: 45 minutes

Servings: 6

Ingredients:

- Swiss cheese (shredded) – 1/2 cup

- Serrano (diced)– 1

- Smoked ham pieces – 2

- Eggs – 1

Directions:

1. Pre-heat waffle iron and grease

2. Fry Smoked ham pieces in a pan

3. Add shredded cheese, egg and serrano and mix together

4. Cook till crisp

Nutrition: Calories 139 Total Fat 4.6 g Total Carbs 2.5 g Sugar 6.3 g Fiber 0.6 g Protein 3.8 g

Crunchy Canadian bacon Chaffles

Preparation Time: 5 minutes

Cooking Time: 5 minutes

Servings: 2

Ingredients:

- Cheddar – 1/3 cup

- Eggs – 1

- Flaxseed (ground) – 1 teaspoon

- Baking powder – 1/4 teaspoon

- Canadian bacon piece – 2 tablespoons

- Parmesan – 1/3 cup

Directions:

1. Cook Canadian bacon in pan

2. Add egg, cheddar cheese, flaxseed and baking powder then mix

3. Shred part of parmesan cheese in waffle iron and grease plate

4. Pour mixture and top with remaining parmesan cheese

5. Cook till crisp

Nutrition: Calories 139 Total Fat 4.6 g Total Carbs 2.5 g Sugar

6.3 g Fiber 0.6 g Protein 3.8 g

Queso Oaxac Tasty Chaffles

Preparation Time: 12 minutes

Cooking Time: 65 minutes

Servings: 8

Ingredients:

- Eggs – 2

- Queso Oaxaca - 1 cup

- Cream cheese – 2 tablespoons

- Coconut flour – 1 teaspoon

- Baking powder – 3/4 tablespoons

- Water (optional) – 2 tablespoons

Directions:

1. Pre-heat waffle iron

2. Put listed ingredients in some bowl and mix

3. Grease waffle iron slightly and cook the mixture in it till crisp

Nutrition: Calories 139 Total Fat 4.6 g Total Carbs 2.5 g Sugar 6.3 g Fiber 0.6 g Protein 3.8 g

Coconut-Olive Chaffles

Preparation Time: 4 minutes

Cooking Time: 10 minutes

Servings: 2

Ingredients:

- Coconut flour – 1 teaspoon

- Eggs – 2

- Water – 2 tablespoons

- Olive oil – 2 tablespoons

- Garlic powder – 1/2 teaspoon

- Baking powder – 1/8 teaspoon

Directi:ons

1. Mix all ingredients in one bowl

2. Preheat waffle iron and lightly grease it

3. Pour mixture and spread evenly

4. Cook till crisp

5. Takes 10 min to prepare and serves 2

Nutrition: Calories 139 Total Fat 4.6 g Total Carbs 2.5 g Sugar 6.3 g Fiber 0.6 g Protein 3.8 g

Swiss Cheese Serrano Chaffles

Preparation Time: 12 minutes

Cooking Time: 30 minutes

Servings: 4

Ingredients

- Eggs – 2

- Swiss cheese – 1 1/2 cups

- Serrano pepper – 10 slices

Directions:

1. Preheat waffle maker

2. Mix eggs and 3/4 cups of Swiss cheese in a bowl

3. Shred Swiss cheese on waffle maker plate

4. Pour mixture onto plate

5. Add cheese on top of mixture

6. Top up with 4 Serrano slices and cook till crunchy

Nutrition: Calories 195 Total Fat 14.3 g Total Carbs 4.5 g Sugar 0.5 g Fiber 0.3 g Protein 3.2 g

MAIN, SIDE & VEGETABLE

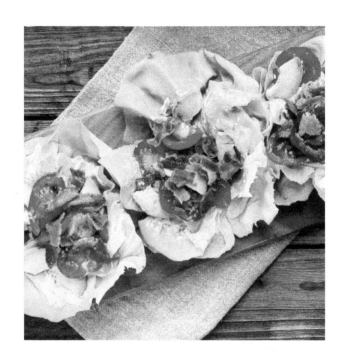

Herb Butter Scallops

Preparation time: 10 minutes

Cooking time: 10 minutes

Servings:3

Ingredients:

- pound sea scallops, cleaned

- Freshly ground black pepper

- 8 tablespoons butter, divided

- teaspoons minced garlic

- Juice of 1 lemon

- teaspoons chopped fresh basil

- teaspoon chopped fresh thyme

Directions:

1.   Pat the scallops dry with paper towels and season them lightly with pepper.

2.   Place a large skillet over medium heat and add 2 tablespoons of butter.

3.   Arrange the scallops in the skillet, evenly spaced but not too close together, and sear each side until they are golden brown, about 2½ minutes per side.

4.   Remove the scallops to a plate and set aside.

5.   Add the remaining 6 tablespoons of butter to the skillet and sauté the garlic until translucent, about 3 minutes.

6.   Stir in the lemon juice, basil, and thyme and return the scallops to the skillet, turning to coat them in the sauce.

7.   Serve immediately.

Nutrition: Calories: 306 Fat: 24g Protein: 19g carbohydrates: 4g Fiber: 0g

Pan-Seared Halibut with Citrus Butter Sauce

Preparation time: 10 minutes

Cooking time: 15 minutes

Servings: 3

Ingredients:

- 4 (5-ounce) halibut fillets, each about 1 inch thick

- Sea salt

- Freshly ground black pepper

- ¼ cup butter

- 2 teaspoons minced garlic

- shallot, minced

- tablespoons dry white wine

- tablespoon freshly squeezed lemon juice

- tablespoon freshly squeezed orange juice

- teaspoons chopped fresh parsley

- tablespoons olive oil

Directions:

1. Pat the fish dry with paper towels and then lightly season the fillets with salt and pepper. Set aside on a paper towel–lined plate.

2. Place a small saucepan over medium heat and melt the butter.

3. Sauté the garlic and shallot until tender, about 3 minutes.

4. Whisk in the white wine, lemon juice, and orange juice and bring the sauce to a simmer, cooking until it thickens slightly, about 2 minutes.

5. Remove the sauce from the heat and stir in the parsley; set aside.

6. Place a large skillet over medium-high heat and add the olive oil.

7. Panfry the fish until lightly browned and just cooked through, turning them over once, about 10 minutes in total.

8. Serve the fish immediately with a spoonful of sauce for each.

Nutrition: Calories: 319 Fat: 26g Protein: 22g Carbohydrates: 2g Fiber: 0g

Cheesy Cauliflower Muffins

Preparation time: 10 minutes

Cooking time: 12 minutes

Servings: 2

Ingredients:

- ¾ cup chopped cauliflower florets

- egg

- ¾ tbsp coconut flour

- ¼ tsp Italian seasoning

- 1/3 cup grated parmesan cheese

- Seasoning:

- ¼ tsp salt

- 1/8 tsp onion powder

- 1/8 tsp garlic powder

Directions:

1.   Turn on the oven, then set it to 375 degrees F and let it preheat.

2.   Take a medium bowl, place chopped cauliflower in it, add flour, half of the cheese, onion powder, garlic powder, and Italian seasoning and stir until incorporated and smooth.

3. Take four silicone cups, fill them with prepared cauliflower mixture, sprinkle remaining cheese on top and then bake for 10 to 12 minutes until thoroughly cooked and firm.

4. Serve.

Nutrition: 77 Calories; 5.6 g Fats; 4.6 g Protein; 1.7 g Net Carb; 0.9 g Fiber;

Pumpkin And Cauliflower Rice

Preparation time: 5 minutes

Cooking time: 10 minutes

Servings: 4

Ingredients:

- 2 ounces olive oil

- yellow onion, chopped

- garlic cloves, minced

- 12 ounces cauliflower rice

- cups chicken stock

- 6 ounces pumpkin puree

- ½ teaspoon nutmeg, ground

- teaspoon thyme chopped

- ½ teaspoon ginger, grated

- ½ teaspoon cinnamon powder

- ½ teaspoon allspice

- ounces coconut cream

Directions:

1.   Set your instant pot on sauté mode, add the oil, heat it up, add garlic and onion, stir and sauté for 3 minutes.

2.   Add cauliflower rice, stock, pumpkin puree, thyme, nutmeg, cinnamon, ginger and allspice, stir, cover and cook on High for 12 minutes.

3.   Add coconut cream, stir, divide among plates and serve as a side dish.

4.   Enjoy!

Nutrition: Calories 152, fat 2, fiber 3, carbs 5, protein 6

Scrambled Eggs with Kale

Preparation time: 5 minutes

Cooking time: 8 minutes

Servings: 2

Ingredients:

- green onion, chopped

- ½ cup chopped kale

- tbsp avocado oil

- eggs

- tbsp grated cheddar cheese

- Seasoning:

- 1/8 tsp garlic powder

- ¼ tsp salt

Directions:

1. Take a medium skillet pan, place it over medium heat, add oil and when hot, add green onion and cook for 1 minute until tender-crisp.

2. Add kale, season with garlic powder and salt, stir until mixed and cook for 1 minute until kale leaves wilt.

3. Crack eggs in a bowl, whisk until well combined, then pour the egg into the pan, spread evenly, and cook for 2 minutes until it begins to set, don't stir.

4. Then scramble the eggs and continue cooking for 2 to 3 minutes until eggs have cooked to the desired level.

5. Sprinkle with cheese and then serve.

Nutrition: 173 Calories; 14.5 g Fats; 8.5 g Protein; 1.2 g Net Carb; 0.1 g Fiber;

Spicy Eggs in Kale

Preparation time: 5 minutes

Cooking time: 10 minutes

Servings: 2

Ingredients:

- bunch of kale

- green onion, sliced

- ½ of lime, juiced, zested

- eggs

- ½ cup chicken broth

- Seasoning:

- 1/3 tsp salt

- 1/4 tsp ground black pepper

- ½ tbsp unsalted butter

Directions:

1.   Take a medium frying pan, place it over medium heat, add butter and when it melts, add onion and cook for 1 minute.

2.   Add kale, cook for 2 minutes until saute, then pour in broth and season with salt and black pepper.

3.   Add lime zest and juice, stir until mixed, pour in chicken broth and simmer for 3 minutes until kale has turned soft.

4.   Switch heat to medium-low level, make two packets in kale, crack an egg into each packet, then cover with the lid and cook for 2 to 3 minutes.

5.   Remove pan from heat, let it rest for 3 minutes, then sprinkle with some black pepper and serve.

Nutrition: 195 Calories; 15.5 g Fats; 9.8 g Protein; 2 g Net Carb; 3 g Fiber;

Simplest Yellow Squash

Preparation Time: 10 minutes

Cooking Time: 12 minutes

Servings: 4

Ingredients:

- 2 tbsp. olive oil

- lb. yellow squash, cut into thin slices

- small yellow onion, cut into thin rings

- garlic clove, minced

- tsp. water

- Salt and freshly ground white pepper, to taste

Directions:

1. In a large skillet, heat the oil over medium-high heat and stir fry the squash, onion and garlic for about 3-4 minutes.

2. Add water, salt and black pepper and stir to combine.

3. Reduce heat to low and simmer for about 6-8 minutes.

4. Serve hot.

Nutrition: Calories: 86; Carbohydrates: 5.7g; Protein: 1.6g; Fat: 7.2g; Sugar: 2.7g; Sodium: 51mg; Fiber: 1.7g

Scallops with Mushroom Special

Preparation Time: 15 minutes

Cooking Time: 20 minutes

Servings: 2

Ingredients:

- lb Scallops

- Onions, chopped

- tbsp Butter

- tbsp Olive oil

- cup Mushrooms

- Salt and Pepper, to taste

- 1 tbsp Lemon juice

- ½ cup Whipping Cream

- 1 tbsp chopped fresh Parsley

Directions:

1. Heat the oil on Sauté. Add onions, butter, mushrooms, salt and pepper. Cook for 3 to 5 minutes. Add the lemon juice and scallops. Lock the lid and set to Manual mode.

2.   Cook for 15 minutes on High pressure. When ready, do a quick pressure release and carefully open the lid. Top with a drizzle of cream and fresh parsley.

Nutrition: Calories 312, Protein 31g, Net Carbs 7.3g, Fat 10.4g

SOUP AND STEWS

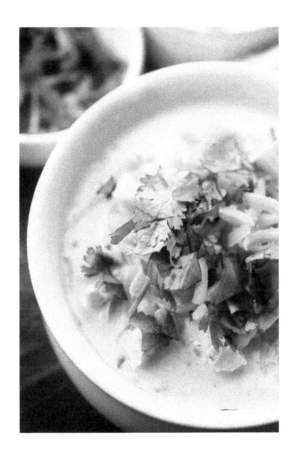

Vegetable Beef Soup

Preparation time: 10 minutes

Cooking time: 4-6 hours

Servings: 6

Ingredients:

- pound lean ground beef

- 4 cups beef broth

- zucchini, diced

- stalks celery, chopped

- ½ cup diced tomatoes

- yellow onion, chopped

- cloves garlic, chopped

- 1 teaspoon freshly chopped thyme

- 1 teaspoon freshly chopped rosemary

- Salt & pepper, to taste

Directions:

1.   Add all the ingredients to a slow cooker and cook on high for 4 to 6 hours.

2.   Stir well before serving.

Nutrition: Calories: 185 Carbs: 5g Fiber: 1g Net Carbs: 4g Fat: 6g Protein: 7g

Hoisin Sauce

Preparation Time: 10 minutes

Cooking Time: 0 minutes

Servings: 8

Ingredients:

• 4 tablespoons low-sodium soy sauce

• 2 tablespoons natural peanut butter

• tablespoon Erythritol

• teaspoons balsamic vinegar

• teaspoons sesame oil

• teaspoon Sriracha

• garlic clove, peeled

• Ground black pepper, as required

Directions:

1. Put all together the ingredients in a food processor and pulse until smooth.

2. You can preserve this sauce in the refrigerator by placing it into an airtight container.

Nutrition: Calories: 39 Net Carbs: 1.2g Carbohydrate: 1.5g Fiber: 0.3g Protein: 1.8g Fat: 3.1g Sugar: 0.8g Sodio

Lamb Taco Soup

Preparation time: 10 minutes

Cooking time: 4-6 hours minutes

Servings: 6

Ingredients:

- pound ground lamb

- 4 cups beef broth

- cup shredded cheddar cheese

- cup diced tomatoes

- 1 green bell pepper, chopped

- 1 yellow onion, chopped

- cloves garlic, chopped

- 1 teaspoon ground cumin

- 1 teaspoon ground coriander

- 1 teaspoon paprika

- ½ teaspoon cayenne pepper

- Salt & pepper, to taste

Directions:

1. Add all the ingredients to a slow cooker minus the shredded cheese and cook on high for 4 to 6 hours.

2.   Stir in the shredded cheese and serve.

Nutrition: Calories: 265 Carbs: 6g Fiber: 1g Net Carbs: 5g Fat: 13g Protein: 30g

Buffalo Sauce

Preparation Time: 10 minutes

Cooking Time: 30 minutes

Servings: 8

Ingredients:

- 8 ounces Cream Cheese (softened)

- ½ cup Buffalo Wing Sauce

- ½ cup Blue Cheese Dressing

- ½ cups Cheddar Cheese (Shredded)

- ¼ cups Chicken Breast (Cooked)

Directions:

1. Preheat oven to 350oF.

2. Blend together the buffalo sauce, white salad dressing, cream cheese, chicken, and shredded cheese.

3. Top with any other optional ingredients like blue cheese chunks.

4. Bake for 25-30 minutes

Nutrition: Calories: 325 Fat: 28g Carbs: 2.2g Protein: 16g

DESSERT

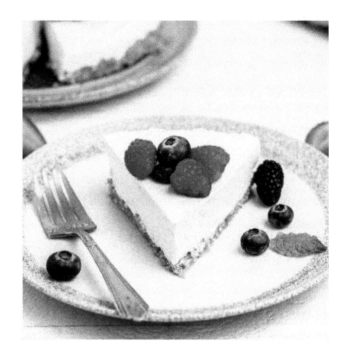

Butter Glazed Cookies

Preparation Time: 15 minutes

Cooking Time: 6 minutes

Servings: 40 cookies

Ingredients:

- 1/3 cup coconut flour

- 2/3 cup almond flour

- 1/4 cup granulated erythritol

- 8 drops stevia

- 1/2 cup butter, softened

- 1 tsp. almond or vanilla extract

- 1/4 tsp. baking powder

- 1/4 tsp. xanthan gum (optional)

- For the Glaze:

- 1/4 cup coconut butter

- 8 drops stevia

Directions:

1. Preheat your oven to 356 degrees F.

2. Whisk dry ingredients in one bowl and beat butter with stevia and vanilla extract in another.

3.   Add dry mixture and mix well until smooth then divide the dough into two pieces.

4.   Place each dough piece in between two sheets of wax paper.

5.   Spread them into a thick sheet and refrigerate for 10 minutes.

6.   Use a cookies cutter to cut small cookies out of both the dough sheets.

7.   Place them on a baking sheet lined with wax paper and bake them for 6 minutes.

8.   Meanwhile, prepare the glaze by heating coconut butter with stevia in a bowl in the microwave.

9.   Pour this glaze over each cookie and allow it to set.

10.   Serve.

Nutrition: Calories 237 Total Fat 22 g Carbs 5 g Sugar 1 g Fiber 2 g Protein 5 g

Chocolate Zucchini Muffins

Preparation Time: 10 minutes

Cooking Time: 30 minutes

Servings: 9

Ingredients:

- 1/2 cup coconut flour

- 3/4 tsp. baking soda

- 2 tbsp. cocoa powder

- 1/2 tsp. salt

- 1 tsp. cinnamon

- 1/2 tsp. nutmeg

- 3 large eggs

- 2/3 cup Swerve sweetener

- 2 tsp. vanilla extract

- 1 tbsp. oil

- 1 medium zucchini, grated

- 1/4 cup heavy cream

- 1/3 cup Lily's chocolate baking chips

Directions:

1. Preheat your oven at 356 degrees F.

2.   Layer a 9-cup o muffin tray with muffin liners then spray them with cooking oil.

3.   Whisk coconut flour with salt, cinnamon, nutmeg, sweetener, baking soda, and cocoa powder in a bowl.

4.   Beat eggs in a separate bowl then add oil, cream, vanilla, and zucchini.

5.   Stir in the coconut flour mixture and mix well until fully incorporated.

6.   Fold in chocolate chips then divide the batter into the lined muffin cups.

7.   Bake these muffins for 30 minutes then allow them to cool on a wire rack.

8.   Enjoy.

Nutrition: Calories 151 Total Fat 14.7 g Total Carbs 1.5 g Sugar 0.3 g Fiber 0.1 g Protein 0.8 g

Chocolate Dipped Cookies

Preparation Time: 10 minutes

Cooking Time: 30 minutes

Servings: 8

Ingredients:

- 1 1/2 cups almond flour

- 1/4 cup almond butter

- 2 tbsp. powdered erythritol

- 1 large egg

- 1 tsp. vanilla powder

- 1 tbsp. virgin coconut oil

- 1 tbsp. coconut butter

- 1 tsp. baking powder

- Pinch of salt

- 1Oz. 90% dark chocolate

Directions:

1. Whisk almond flour, vanilla, salt, baking powder, and erythritol in a mixing bowl.

2. Stir in almond butter, egg, coconut butter, and coconut oil.

3. Mix well to form a dough then place it in a sandwich bag. Refrigerate for 30 minutes.

4. Let your oven preheat at 285 degrees F.

5. Place the dough in between two sheets of parchment then roll it into a 1/2-inch thick sheet.

6. Use a 2.5-inch diameter cookie cutter to cut the cookies out of this dough.

7. Reroll the remaining dough then place it on a greased baking sheet.

8. Bake the cookies for 30 minutes until golden brown.

9. Place them on a wire rack to cool down.

10. Melt chocolate in a bowl by heating in a microwave and stir well.

11. Dip half of each cooled cookie in the chocolate melt and allow it to set on wax paper.

12. Refrigerate the dipped cookies for 15 minutes.

13. Serve.

Nutrition: Calories 236 Total Fat 13.5 g Total Carbs 1.6 g Sugar 1.4 g Fiber 3.8 g Protein 4.3 g

Mint Creme Oreos

Preparation Time: 10 minutes

Cooking Time: 12 minutes

Servings: 12

Ingredients:

- 2 1/4 cups almond flour

- 3 tbsp. coconut flour

- 4 tbsp. cacao powder

- 1 tsp. baking powder

- 1 1/2 tsp. xanthan gum

- 1/4 tsp. salt

- 1/2 cup grass-fed butter, unsalted and softened

- 1 egg

- 1 tsp. vanilla extract

- 4 oz. cream cheese

- 1 cup lakanto monk fruit

- 1 tsp. peppermint extract

Directions:

1. Preheat your oven to 350 degrees F.

2. Mix coconut flour with almond flour, xanthan gum, salt, baking powder, and cocoa powder in a medium-sized bowl.

3. Whisk 1/2 cup monk fruit sweetener with six tablespoons of butter in a bowl until fluffy.

4. Add vanilla extract and egg then beat well and stir in dry ingredients to form the dough.

5. Place this dough in between two sheets of wax paper and roll it into a 1/8-inch thick sheet.

6. Cut cookies with a round cookie cutter then re-roll the remaining dough to cut more cookies.

7. Place these cookies on a cookie sheet lined with parchment paper.

8. Bake these cookies for 12 minutes then allow them to cool.

9. Meanwhile, beat cream cheese with 2 tablespoons butter, 1/2 cup monk fruit, and peppermint extract in a small bowl.

10. Divide this mixture over half of the cookies.

11. Place the remaining half of the cookies over the cream filling.

12.   Press the two halves together gently.

13.   Enjoy.

Nutrition: Calories 331 Total Fat 12.9 g Carbs 1.1 g Sugar 2.8 g

Fiber 0.8 g Protein 4.4 g

Blackberry-Filled Lemon Muffins

Preparation Time: 5 minutes

Cooking Time: 30 minutes

Servings: 12

Ingredients:

- For the Blackberry Filling:

- 3 tbsp granulated stevia

- 1 tsp lemon juice

- 1/4 tsp xanthan gum

- 2 tbsp water

- 1 cup fresh blackberries

- For the Muffin Batter:

- 2 1/2 cups super fine almond flour

- 3/4 cup granulasted stevia

- 1 tsp fresh lemon zest

- 1/2 tsp sea salt

- 1 tsp grain-free baking powder

- 4 large eggs

- 1/4 cup unsweetened almond milk

- 1/4 cup butter

- 1 tsp vanilla extract

- 1/2 tsp lemon extract

Directions:

1. For the Blackberry Filling:

2. Add granulated sweetener and xanthan gum in a saucepan.

3. Stir in lemon juice and water then place it over the medium heat.

4. Add blackberries and stir cook on low heat for 10 minutes.

5. Remove the saucepan from the heat and allow the mixture to cool.

6. For the Muffin Batter:

7. Preheat your oven at 356 degrees F and layer a muffin tray with paper cups.

8. Mix almond flour with salt, baking powder, lemon zest, baking powder, and sweetener in a mixing bowl.

9. Whisk in eggs, vanilla extract, lemon extract, butter, and almond milk.

10.   Beat well until smooth. Divide half of this batter into the muffin tray.

11.   Make a depression at the center of each muffin.

12.   Add a spoonful of blackberry jam mixture to each depression.

13.   Cover the filling with remaining batter on top.

14.   Bake the muffins for 30 minutes then allow them to cool.

15.   Refrigerate for a few hours before serving.

16.   Enjoy.

Nutrition: Calories 261 Total Fat 7.1 g Total Carbs 3.1 g Sugar 2.1 g Fiber 3.9 g Protein 1.8 g

Shortbread Cookies

Preparation Time: 10 minutes

Cooking Time: 13 minutes

Servings: 6

Ingredients:

- 1 1/2 cups almond flour

- 1/2 tsp. xanthan gum

- 1/4 tsp. kosher salt

- 6 tbsp. grass-fed butter, room temperature

- 6 tbsp. powdered erythritol

- 1/2 tsp. vanilla extract

Directions:

1.   Spread almond flour in a dry skillet and place it over medium heat.

2.   Stir cook for 3 minutes or more until golden brown then remove it from the heat.

3.   Add salt and xanthan gum to the flour and mix well.

4.   Beat butter with an electric mixer for 3 minutes and add sweetener.

5. Continue beating then add vanilla extract. Beat until combined.

6. Add almond flour mixture and whisk well until it forms a smooth dough.

7. Wrap the dough in a plastic wrap then refrigerate for 1 hour.

8. Let your oven preheat at 350 degrees F and grease a baking tray with cooking oil.

9. Place the cookie dough between two parchment sheets and roll it into a 1/4-inch thick sheet.

10. Cut out cookies using any shape cookie cutter.

11. Arrange all the cookies on a baking sheet and freeze for 15 minutes.

12. Bake them for 13 minutes until golden brown.

13. Serve.

Nutrition: Calories 167 Total Fat 5.1 G Total Carbs 1.9 G Sugar 3.8 G Fiber 2.1 G Protein 6.3 G

Peanut Butter Cookies

Preparation Time: 20 minutes

Cooking Time: 36 minutes

Servings: 12

Ingredients

- 1/2 cup peanut butter

- 1/2 cup powdered erythritol

- 1 egg

Directions:

1. Preheat your oven to 350 degrees F.

2. Layer a baking sheet with wax paper and set it aside.

3. Add all the ingredients to a bowl and mix well to prepare the cookie dough.

4. Add 1.5 tablespoons of the dough on the baking sheet scoop by scoop to make the cookies.

5. Bake for 15 minutes until golden brown.

6. Enjoy.

Nutrition: 55 Calories; 3.5 g Fats; 4.5 g Protein; 0.4 g Net Carb; 0.2 g Fiber;

Lightning Source UK Ltd.
Milton Keynes UK
UKHW020849180521
383917UK00001B/64